You Can Lose Weight

Welcome to "You Can Lose Weight," a comprehensive guide to sustainable weight loss that transcends the limitations of quick fixes and crash diets. In these pages, we embark on a journey together—a journey towards understanding the complexities of weight loss, embracing evidence-based strategies for long-term success, and cultivating a mindset of empowerment, resilience, and self-compassion.

Drawing upon the latest research in nutrition, exercise science, psychology, and holistic wellness, this book offers a roadmap for navigating the challenges and opportunities of the weight loss journey. From setting realistic goals and understanding the science of metabolism to exploring diverse dietary approaches and embracing holistic self-care practices, each chapter is designed to empower you with the knowledge, tools, and confidence to achieve lasting transformation from the inside out.

But this book is more than just a roadmap— it's a companion, a coach, and a source of inspiration and support as you embark on this transformative journey. Through personal anecdotes, expert insights, and practical advice, we'll explore not only the physical aspects of weight loss but also the emotional, psychological, and spiritual dimensions of reclaiming your health and vitality.

As you delve into the pages of "You Can Lose Weight," I invite you to approach this journey with an open mind, a compassionate heart, and a willingness to embrace change. Together, we'll challenge conventional wisdom, break free from limiting beliefs, and chart a course towards a future of health, happiness, and fulfillment that surpasses your wildest dreams.

Whether you're just beginning your weight loss journey or seeking to reignite your motivation and momentum, this book is here to guide and support you every step of the way. So let's embark on this transformative journey together, and let's discover the power within you to transform your body, transform your life, and create the vibrant, fulfilling future you deserve.

Contents

Chapter 1: Introduction to Modern Weight Loss

Understanding the Current Landscape: Insights into the challenges and opportunities of weight loss

In the ever-evolving landscape of health and wellness, the pursuit of weight loss stands as one of the most enduring and universal goals. However, the approach to weight loss has undergone a significant transformation. Gone are the days of one-size-fits-all solutions and crash diets promising miraculous results. Instead, we find ourselves amidst a revolution in understanding, fueled by science, technology, and a holistic approach to well-being.

The traditional narrative surrounding weight loss often centered solely on calorie counting and intense exercise regimens. While these factors remain essential, modern weight loss acknowledges that the journey to a healthier weight encompasses far more than simple arithmetic and sweat. It recognizes the interconnectedness of physical, mental, and emotional health, and the importance of addressing the root causes of weight gain rather than merely treating the symptoms.

One of the most significant shifts in the paradigm of weight loss is the emphasis on personalized approaches. No longer do we subscribe to generic, one-size-fits-all plans that fail to account for individual differences in biology, lifestyle, and preferences. Instead, we recognize the importance of tailoring strategies to suit each person's unique needs, goals, and circumstances. Whether it's finding the right balance of macronutrients, identifying enjoyable forms of physical activity, or addressing underlying psychological barriers, modern weight loss is all about customization and empowerment.

Moreover, advancements in scientific research have shed new light on the complexities of metabolism, genetics, and the gut microbiome, offering insights that were previously unimaginable. We now understand that weight management is not solely a matter of willpower but is influenced by a myriad of factors, including hormonal balance, sleep quality, stress levels, and environmental cues. Armed with this knowledge, we are better equipped to design comprehensive, evidence-based strategies that foster sustainable weight loss and long-term health.

Furthermore, technology has emerged as a powerful ally in the quest for weight loss success. From smartphone apps that track food intake and monitor physical activity to wearable devices that provide real-time feedback and motivation, the digital revolution has democratized access to tools and resources that were once reserved for elite athletes and celebrities. These innovations not only make it easier to stay accountable and track progress but also facilitate greater connectivity and support within communities of like-minded individuals.

In this brave new world of weight loss, we also recognize the importance of addressing the psychological and emotional aspects of the journey. Long gone are the days of shame and stigma surrounding body size, replaced instead by a culture of self-compassion, body positivity, and empowerment. We understand that true transformation begins from within, requiring not only changes in behavior but also shifts in mindset and self-perception.

As we embark on this journey together, let us embrace the principles of modern weight loss:

empowerment, customization, evidence-based practice, and holistic well-being. Let us celebrate the diversity of paths that lead to a healthier weight and honor the resilience and determination of every individual who dares to embark on this transformative journey. Welcome to the dawn of a new era in weight loss, where the possibilities are as boundless as our collective determination to thrive.

The Science of Weight Loss: Delving into the latest research and understanding the body's mechanisms for shedding pounds.

In the pursuit of weight loss, knowledge is power. Understanding the intricate workings of the human body and how it responds to various stimuli is key to devising effective strategies for shedding pounds and maintaining a healthy weight. In this chapter, we delve into the latest scientific research to uncover the underlying mechanisms of weight loss and explore evidence-based approaches for achieving lasting results.

At its core, weight loss is a matter of energy balance: calories consumed versus calories expended. However, the body's response to this energy imbalance is far more complex than a simple mathematical equation. Numerous physiological processes come into play, influencing everything from appetite and metabolism to fat storage and utilization.

One of the primary determinants of weight loss is the metabolic rate, or the rate at which the body burns calories to sustain basic physiological functions. While genetics play a role in determining metabolic rate, lifestyle factors such as diet, exercise, and sleep quality also exert significant influence. By adopting a balanced diet rich in nutrient-dense foods, engaging in regular physical activity, and prioritizing adequate sleep, individuals can optimize their metabolic rate and support their weight loss efforts.

Another key player in the science of weight loss is the hormone leptin, often referred to as the "satiety hormone." Produced by fat cells, leptin helps regulate appetite and energy expenditure by signaling to the brain when the body has had enough to eat. However, in cases of obesity, leptin resistance can occur, leading to a dysregulation of appetite control and contributing to overeating and weight gain. Understanding the role of leptin and strategies for enhancing leptin sensitivity can be instrumental in promoting successful weight loss.

Furthermore, research has shed new light on the role of the gut microbiome—the vast ecosystem of microorganisms that inhabit the digestive tract—in weight regulation. Emerging evidence suggests that certain strains of gut bacteria may influence metabolism, appetite, and fat storage, offering potential targets for interventions aimed at promoting weight loss. By consuming a diverse array of fiber-rich foods and probiotic-rich fermented foods, individuals can support the health of their gut microbiome and potentially enhance their weight loss efforts.

In addition to these physiological factors, the psychological and emotional aspects of weight loss cannot be overlooked. Stress, depression, and other mental health conditions can significantly impact eating behaviors and weight management outcomes. By addressing underlying psychological barriers and cultivating mindfulness, self-awareness, and stress management techniques, individuals can bolster their resilience and improve their chances of long-term success.

In summary, the science of weight loss is a multifaceted and dynamic field, encompassing a wide range of physiological, psychological, and environmental factors. By staying abreast of the latest research and understanding the body's mechanisms for shedding pounds, individuals can make informed decisions and adopt evidence-based strategies that promote sustainable weight loss and overall well-being.

Setting Realistic Goals: Crafting achievable objectives tailored to individual needs and lifestyles.

Embarking on a journey towards weight loss is often accompanied by a surge of motivation and determination. However, sustaining that momentum over the long term requires more than just sheer willpower—it necessitates setting realistic and achievable goals that align with one's individual needs and lifestyle. In this chapter, we explore the importance of goal-setting in the context of weight loss and provide guidance on how to craft objectives that foster success and sustainability.

The foundation of effective goal-setting lies in its specificity and attainability. Rather than vague aspirations such as "losing weight" or "getting in shape," individuals benefit from defining clear, measurable, and actionable goals that are tailored to their unique circumstances. Whether it's aiming to lose a certain number of pounds, fitting into a specific clothing size, or improving physical fitness levels, specificity provides a roadmap for progress and helps individuals stay focused and accountable.

Moreover, setting realistic goals entails taking into account one's current lifestyle, commitments, and constraints. While ambitious goals may be inspiring, they can quickly become demoralizing if they are not aligned with practical considerations such as time, resources, and other obligations. By considering factors such as work schedules, family responsibilities, and social commitments, individuals can set themselves up for success by establishing goals that are challenging yet attainable within their existing framework.

Furthermore, goals should be framed in a positive and empowering manner, focusing on what individuals can achieve rather than what they need to eliminate or restrict. For example, instead of setting a goal to "stop eating junk food," reframing it as a goal to "incorporate more whole, nutrient-dense foods into meals and snacks" fosters a mindset of abundance and empowerment rather than deprivation.

In addition to setting long-term goals, it is essential to break them down into smaller, manageable milestones that can be celebrated along the way. By establishing short-term objectives that build upon each other, individuals can maintain motivation and momentum as they progress towards their ultimate goal. Celebrating these milestones, whether it's reaching a certain weight milestone, mastering a new exercise routine, or consistently adhering to a healthy eating plan, reinforces positive behaviors and fosters a sense of accomplishment.

Furthermore, flexibility is key to successful goal-setting, as circumstances may change, and setbacks are inevitable. Rather than viewing setbacks as failures, individuals can use them as opportunities for learning and growth, adjusting their goals and strategies as needed to continue moving forward. By cultivating a growth mindset and embracing the journey as a process of continuous improvement, individuals can navigate challenges with resilience and optimism.

In summary, setting realistic goals is a critical component of achieving success in weight loss endeavors. By crafting objectives that are

specific, attainable, and aligned with one's
individual needs and lifestyle, individuals can
lay the groundwork for sustainable progress
and long-term success. With clarity, positivity,
and flexibility, each step towards achieving
these goals becomes a meaningful milestone
on the path to a healthier, happier life.

Chapter 2: Navigating the Dietary Maze

Trending Diets: From keto to intermittent fasting, exploring popular dietary strategies and their efficacy.

In the ever-evolving landscape of nutrition and weight loss, trending diets often capture the spotlight, promising rapid results and transformative effects on health and well-being. From ketogenic diets to intermittent fasting regimens, each dietary approach comes with its own set of principles, rules, and purported benefits. In this chapter, we delve into some of the most popular trending diets, exploring their efficacy, potential benefits, and considerations for implementation.

1. Ketogenic Diet (Keto):
   The ketogenic diet is a high-fat, low-carbohydrate eating plan designed to induce a state of ketosis, wherein the body shifts from using glucose as its primary fuel source to burning fat for energy. By severely restricting

carbohydrates and increasing fat intake, the keto diet aims to promote weight loss, improve metabolic health, and enhance cognitive function. While research suggests that the keto diet may be effective for short-term weight loss and managing certain medical conditions such as epilepsy and type 2 diabetes, its long-term sustainability and potential risks, such as nutrient deficiencies and adverse lipid profiles, remain subjects of debate among health experts.

2. Intermittent Fasting (IF):

Intermittent fasting encompasses various eating patterns that cycle between periods of fasting and eating. Common IF protocols include the 16/8 method (fasting for 16 hours and eating within an 8-hour window), the 5:2 diet (eating normally for five days and restricting calories on two non-consecutive days), and alternate-day fasting (alternating between fasting and regular eating days). Advocates of intermittent fasting tout its potential benefits for weight loss, insulin sensitivity, and cellular repair processes. While research suggests that IF may offer metabolic benefits and aid in weight management, individual responses can vary, and long-term adherence may pose challenges for some individuals.

3. Plant-Based Diet:

Plant-based diets emphasize whole, minimally processed plant foods such as fruits, vegetables, whole grains, legumes, nuts, and seeds while limiting or excluding animal products. Research indicates that plant-based diets may offer numerous health benefits, including weight management, improved heart health, reduced risk of chronic diseases, and enhanced longevity. By focusing on nutrient-dense plant foods, plant-based diets provide ample fiber, vitamins, minerals, and antioxidants while minimizing intake of saturated fat and cholesterol. However, it's essential to ensure adequate intake of key nutrients such as protein, iron, calcium, vitamin B12, and omega-3 fatty acids when following a plant-based diet, particularly for those who exclude all animal products.

4. Mediterranean Diet:

The Mediterranean diet is inspired by the traditional eating patterns of countries bordering the Mediterranean Sea, characterized by an abundance of fruits, vegetables, whole grains, legumes, nuts, seeds, olive oil, fish, and moderate consumption of poultry, eggs, and dairy. The Mediterranean diet is renowned for its potential to promote heart health, reduce inflammation, and support weight management. Rich in fiber, antioxidants, monounsaturated fats, and omega-3 fatty acids, this dietary pattern emphasizes whole, minimally processed foods while minimizing intake of red meat, processed foods, and added sugars.

While each of these trending diets offers unique principles and potential benefits, it's essential to approach dietary changes with careful consideration of individual needs, preferences, and health goals. Consulting with a qualified healthcare professional or registered dietitian can provide personalized guidance and support in navigating the complexities of nutrition and weight management. Ultimately, the most effective dietary approach is one that is sustainable, balanced, and tailored to meet the individual needs and preferences of each person.

The Power of Nutrition: Learning to make informed choices, decode food labels, and optimize nutrient intake.

Nutrition serves as the foundation of health and vitality, influencing every aspect of our well-being, from energy levels and mood to disease risk and longevity. In a world inundated with food choices and conflicting messages, understanding the power of nutrition is essential for making informed decisions that support optimal health. In this chapter, we explore the importance of nutrition, strategies for decoding food labels, and tips for optimizing nutrient intake.

1. Understanding Macronutrients:

- *Macronutrients*—carbohydrates, proteins, and fats—are the building blocks of our diet, providing the energy and nutrients needed for bodily functions. Each macronutrient plays a distinct role in the body:

- *Carbohydrates*: Serve as the primary source of energy, found in foods such as fruits, vegetables, grains, and legumes.

- *Proteins*: Essential for building and repairing tissues, synthesizing enzymes and hormones, and supporting immune function, found in foods such as meat, poultry, fish, eggs, dairy, legumes, nuts, and seeds.

- *Fats*: Provide energy, support cell growth, protect organs, and aid in the absorption of fat-soluble vitamins, found in foods such as avocados, nuts, seeds, olive oil, fatty fish, and dairy products.

2. Decoding Food Labels:

Food labels provide valuable information about the nutritional content of packaged foods, enabling consumers to make informed choices. Key components of food labels include:

- *Serving Size*: Indicates the recommended serving size and the number of servings per container.

- *Calories*: Provides the number of calories per serving, helping individuals manage their energy intake.

- *Nutrient Content*: Lists the amounts of various nutrients (e.g., fat, carbohydrates, protein, vitamins, minerals) per serving, expressed in grams or percentages of daily values (%DV).

- *Ingredients List*: Enumerates the ingredients used in the product, arranged in descending order by weight.

3. Optimizing Nutrient Intake:
- *Emphasize Whole, Nutrient-Dense Foods*: Prioritize whole foods such as fruits, vegetables, whole grains, lean proteins, and healthy fats, which are rich in essential nutrients and fiber.

- *Practice Portion Control*: Be mindful of portion sizes to avoid overeating and support weight management goals.

   - *Balance Macronutrients*: Aim for a balanced intake of carbohydrates, proteins, and fats to meet daily energy needs and support overall health.

   - *Choose Quality Over Quantity*: Opt for minimally processed foods and limit consumption of highly processed, sugary, and high-fat foods that offer little nutritional value.

   - *Stay Hydrated*: Drink plenty of water throughout the day to maintain hydration and support optimal bodily functions.

By honing the skills to make informed choices, decode food labels, and optimize nutrient intake, individuals can harness the power of nutrition to fuel their bodies, enhance their well-being, and achieve their health goals. Whether striving for weight loss, improved energy levels, or disease prevention, adopting a balanced and mindful approach to nutrition lays the groundwork for a lifetime of vitality and resilience.

Mindful Eating: Techniques for cultivating a healthier relationship with food and avoiding emotional eating triggers.

In a culture dominated by busy schedules, distractions, and on-the-go eating, the practice of mindful eating offers a powerful antidote, inviting individuals to reconnect with their bodies, senses, and relationship with food. By bringing awareness and intention to the eating experience, mindful eating promotes greater satisfaction, enjoyment, and balance, while also helping individuals recognize and manage emotional eating triggers. In this chapter, we explore techniques for cultivating mindful eating habits and fostering a healthier relationship with food.

1. Presence and Awareness:

Mindful eating begins with cultivating a sense of presence and awareness during meals and snacks. Rather than rushing through meals or eating mindlessly while distracted, individuals can bring attention to the sensory experience of eating, including sight, smell, taste, texture, and even the sounds of chewing. By slowing down and savoring each bite, individuals can fully engage with the eating process and derive greater pleasure and satisfaction from their meals.

2. Tuning into Hunger and Fullness Cues:

Mindful eating encourages individuals to tune into their body's hunger and fullness cues, rather than relying on external cues or emotional triggers to dictate when and how much to eat. By paying attention to physical sensations of hunger and satiety, individuals can honor their body's natural signals and eat in accordance with their true nutritional needs. Techniques such as the hunger scale, which rates hunger and fullness on a scale from 1 to 10, can help individuals develop greater awareness of their body's cues and avoid overeating or undereating.

3. Emotional Awareness and Regulation:

Emotional eating—eating in response to emotions rather than physical hunger—is a common phenomenon that can interfere with healthy eating habits and weight management goals. Mindful eating encourages individuals to cultivate greater emotional awareness and regulation, allowing them to recognize and respond to emotional triggers without turning to food for comfort or distraction. Techniques such as mindful breathing, meditation, and journaling can help individuals develop healthier coping mechanisms for managing stress, anxiety, boredom, and other emotional states.

4. Non-Judgmental Acceptance:

Mindful eating emphasizes a non-judgmental and compassionate attitude towards oneself and one's eating habits. Rather than viewing certain foods as "good" or "bad" or attaching moral value to eating behaviors, individuals are encouraged to approach food with curiosity, openness, and self-compassion. By releasing guilt, shame, and self-criticism around food choices, individuals can foster a more positive and sustainable relationship with eating, free from restrictive dieting mentality and disordered eating patterns.

5. Mindful Meal Planning and Preparation:

Mindful eating extends beyond the act of eating itself to include meal planning and preparation. By thoughtfully selecting and preparing foods that nourish the body and satisfy the senses, individuals can enhance the eating experience and promote greater enjoyment and satisfaction. Techniques such as mindful grocery shopping, meal prepping with intention, and cooking with mindfulness can deepen one's connection to food and support healthier eating habits overall.

By incorporating these techniques into daily life, individuals can cultivate a more mindful approach to eating, fostering greater awareness, satisfaction, and balance in their relationship with food. Whether seeking to manage weight, improve eating habits, or enhance overall well-being, mindful eating offers a transformative pathway to greater nourishment, self-awareness, and joy in the eating experience.

Chapter 3: Exercise Evolution

Beyond the Gym: Embracing diverse physical activities, from HIIT workouts to outdoor adventures and virtual fitness experiences.

Physical activity is an essential pillar of a healthy lifestyle, offering numerous benefits for both body and mind. While the traditional gym setting has long been synonymous with exercise, there exists a vast and diverse array of physical activities that can contribute to overall fitness, enjoyment, and well-being. In this chapter, we explore the concept of "beyond the gym," highlighting alternative forms of exercise, from high-intensity interval training (HIIT) workouts to outdoor adventures and virtual fitness experiences.

1. High-Intensity Interval Training (HIIT):
   HIIT workouts have gained popularity in recent years for their time-efficient and effective approach to fitness. HIIT involves alternating between short bursts of intense exercise and brief periods of rest or lower-

intensity activity. This style of training can be adapted to various forms of exercise, including running, cycling, strength training, and bodyweight exercises. HIIT workouts are known for their ability to improve cardiovascular health, increase metabolism, and enhance muscular strength and endurance in a shorter amount of time compared to traditional steady-state cardio workouts.

2. Outdoor Adventures:

Engaging in outdoor activities offers a refreshing alternative to indoor exercise, allowing individuals to connect with nature while reaping the benefits of physical activity. Whether it's hiking, biking, kayaking, rock climbing, or simply taking a leisurely walk in the park, outdoor adventures provide opportunities to challenge the body, stimulate the senses, and nourish the soul. Outdoor activities offer a change of scenery, fresh air, and exposure to natural elements, which can invigorate the mind and enhance overall well-being.

3. Group Fitness Classes:

Group fitness classes provide a supportive and motivating environment for individuals to engage in structured workouts led by certified instructors. From dance-based cardio classes to strength training sessions and yoga flows, group fitness classes offer a diverse range of options to suit different interests and fitness levels. The camaraderie and sense of community fostered in group settings can boost motivation, accountability, and enjoyment, making exercise feel more like a social event than a chore.

4. Virtual Fitness Experiences:

In recent years, the rise of technology has paved the way for virtual fitness experiences, allowing individuals to access workouts and classes from the comfort of their own home. Whether through live-streamed classes, on-demand workout videos, or interactive fitness apps, virtual fitness platforms offer convenience, flexibility, and variety. Virtual workouts enable individuals to customize their exercise routines, access expert guidance, and connect with a global community of like-minded individuals, regardless of location or schedule constraints.

5. Mind-Body Practices:

Beyond traditional forms of exercise, mind-body practices such as yoga, Pilates, tai chi, and qigong offer holistic approaches to fitness and well-being. These practices emphasize the integration of breath, movement, and mindfulness to promote physical, mental, and emotional balance. Mind-body practices can improve flexibility, strength, and posture while reducing stress, anxiety, and tension. Whether practiced individually or in a group setting, mind-body exercises provide opportunities for self-reflection, relaxation, and inner exploration.

In summary, "beyond the gym" encompasses a diverse and dynamic spectrum of physical activities that cater to individual preferences, interests, and lifestyles. By embracing alternative forms of exercise such as HIIT workouts, outdoor adventures, group fitness classes, virtual fitness experiences, and mind-body practices, individuals can enrich their fitness journey, discover new passions, and cultivate a lifelong commitment to health and well-being. Whether breaking a sweat in the great outdoors, flowing through a yoga sequence at home, or pushing limits in a high-intensity interval workout, the possibilities for movement and exploration are endless.

Tech Tools for Fitness: Leveraging wearable devices, fitness apps, and virtual trainers to enhance motivation and track progress.

In the digital age, technology has revolutionized the way we approach fitness and exercise, offering a plethora of tools and resources to support our health and wellness goals. From wearable devices and fitness apps to virtual trainers and online communities, tech tools have empowered individuals to take control of their fitness journey, stay motivated, and track their progress with precision and convenience. In this chapter, we explore the various ways in which technology is transforming the fitness landscape and empowering individuals to achieve their fitness aspirations.

1. Wearable Devices:

Wearable fitness trackers, such as smartwatches, fitness bands, and activity monitors, have become increasingly popular for monitoring physical activity, tracking workouts, and measuring key health metrics. These devices typically offer features such as step counting, heart rate monitoring, sleep tracking, calorie expenditure estimation, and GPS tracking for outdoor activities. By providing real-time feedback and insights into their activity levels, wearable devices can motivate individuals to stay active, set goals, and monitor their progress over time.

2. Fitness Apps:

Fitness apps offer a wide range of features and functionalities to support various aspects of health and fitness, from workout planning and tracking to nutrition guidance and mindfulness practices. These apps may include workout libraries with instructional videos, customizable training plans, progress tracking tools, meal planners, calorie counters, and social support networks. Whether looking to build strength, improve cardiovascular fitness, or cultivate mindfulness, fitness apps provide personalized guidance and support to help individuals achieve their goals.

3. Virtual Trainers:

Virtual trainers and online coaching programs offer personalized fitness guidance and support from certified trainers and fitness professionals, delivered through digital platforms such as websites, apps, and video conferencing. Virtual trainers may offer one-on-one coaching sessions, customized workout plans, nutritional guidance, and accountability support to help individuals stay on track and achieve their fitness goals. By leveraging technology, virtual trainers can provide flexible and convenient solutions for individuals seeking expert guidance and motivation on their fitness journey.

4. Gamification and Challenges:

Many fitness apps and wearable devices incorporate elements of gamification, such as challenges, rewards, and leaderboards, to enhance motivation and engagement. These gamified features encourage individuals to set goals, compete with friends, earn badges or points, and celebrate achievements along the way. By turning fitness into a fun and interactive experience, gamification can increase adherence to exercise routines and foster a sense of community and camaraderie among users.

5. Data Analysis and Insights:

One of the most powerful aspects of technology in fitness is its ability to collect, analyze, and interpret data to provide insights into one's health and fitness progress. Wearable devices and fitness apps often offer detailed analytics and reports on metrics such as activity levels, heart rate variability, sleep quality, and workout intensity. By leveraging this data, individuals can gain a deeper understanding of their habits, identify areas for improvement, and make informed decisions to optimize their fitness journey.

In summary, tech tools for fitness offer a wealth of opportunities to enhance motivation, track progress, and achieve fitness goals with greater precision and convenience than ever before. Whether through wearable devices, fitness apps, virtual trainers, or gamified challenges, individuals have access to a diverse array of resources to support their health and wellness aspirations. By harnessing the power of technology and embracing innovation in fitness, individuals can embark on a journey towards greater vitality, strength, and well-being.

Incorporating Movement into Daily Life: Strategies for staying active amidst busy schedules and sedentary environments.

In today's fast-paced world, finding time for regular exercise can be challenging, especially when faced with demanding work schedules, family commitments, and sedentary environments. However, staying active is essential for maintaining physical health, managing stress, and promoting overall well-being. Fortunately, there are many strategies for incorporating movement into daily life, even amidst busy schedules and sedentary lifestyles. In this chapter, we explore practical

tips and techniques for staying active
throughout the day.

1. Prioritize Physical Activity:

Making physical activity a priority is the first
step towards incorporating movement into
daily life. Schedule regular exercise sessions
into your calendar, treating them as non-
negotiable appointments with yourself.
Whether it's a morning jog, a lunchtime yoga
class, or an evening walk, carving out
dedicated time for movement helps ensure
consistency and accountability.

2. Break Up Sedentary Time:

Combatting sedentary behavior is crucial for
overall health, especially for those with desk-
bound jobs or long periods of screen time.
Break up prolonged periods of sitting by
incorporating short movement breaks
throughout the day. Set a timer to remind
yourself to stand up, stretch, or take a brief
walk every hour. Even a few minutes of
movement can help improve circulation,
reduce muscle tension, and boost energy
levels.

3. Find Opportunities to Move:

Look for opportunities to incorporate movement into everyday activities, such as taking the stairs instead of the elevator, parking further away from your destination, or walking or biking for short errands instead of driving. Use household chores as an opportunity to get moving, such as vacuuming, gardening, or cleaning, which can burn calories and contribute to daily activity levels.

4. Make it Enjoyable:

Find activities that you genuinely enjoy and look forward to, as this will increase your motivation to stay active. Experiment with different forms of exercise until you find what resonates with you, whether it's dancing, swimming, hiking, or playing a team sport. Incorporating movement into daily life becomes much easier when it feels less like a chore and more like a source of enjoyment and fulfillment.

5. Involve Others:

Incorporating movement into daily life can be more fun and motivating when shared with others. Invite friends, family members, or colleagues to join you for a walk, hike, or workout session. Participating in group activities or classes can provide social support, accountability, and encouragement, making it easier to stay committed to your fitness goals.

6. Be Creative and Flexible:

Don't be afraid to get creative and think outside the box when it comes to staying active. Take advantage of opportunities to move in unexpected ways, such as dancing while cooking dinner, doing bodyweight exercises during TV commercial breaks, or practicing yoga or stretching before bed. Be flexible and adaptable, adjusting your activity levels based on your schedule, energy levels, and preferences.

In summary, incorporating movement into daily life is not only feasible but essential for maintaining overall health and well-being, even amidst busy schedules and sedentary environments. By prioritizing physical activity, breaking up sedentary time, finding enjoyable activities, involving others, and staying flexible and creative, individuals can cultivate a more active lifestyle and reap the countless benefits of regular exercise. Remember that every little bit of movement counts, so seize every opportunity to get up, get moving, and thrive in a more active way of life.

Chapter 4: The Psychology of Weight Loss

Overcoming Mental Blocks: Addressing common barriers such as self-doubt, fear of failure, and negative self-talk.

Embarking on a journey towards health and fitness is not just about physical activity and nutrition—it also involves navigating the mental and emotional terrain that can often impede progress and hinder success. Mental blocks such as self-doubt, fear of failure, and negative self-talk can sabotage efforts towards adopting healthier habits and achieving fitness goals. In this chapter, we explore strategies for overcoming these common barriers and cultivating a mindset of resilience, confidence, and self-compassion.

1. Recognize and Challenge Negative Thoughts:
   The first step in overcoming mental blocks is to become aware of the negative thoughts and beliefs that may be holding you back. Pay attention to the inner dialogue running

through your mind and identify any patterns
of self-doubt, fear, or self-criticism. Once
identified, challenge these negative thoughts
by asking yourself if they are based on facts or
assumptions, and replace them with more
positive and empowering affirmations.

2. Cultivate Self-Compassion:

Treat yourself with the same kindness and
understanding that you would offer to a friend
facing similar challenges. Recognize that
setbacks and obstacles are a natural part of
the journey towards health and fitness, and
respond to yourself with compassion and
encouragement rather than harsh judgment
or criticism. Practice self-care activities such
as meditation, journaling, or spending time in
nature to nurture your emotional well-being
and build resilience in the face of adversity.

3. Set Realistic Expectations:

Unrealistic expectations can set you up for
disappointment and frustration, leading to
feelings of failure and self-doubt. Instead, set
achievable goals that are within your control
and aligned with your current circumstances
and abilities. Break larger goals into smaller,
manageable steps, and celebrate each
milestone along the way. By focusing on
progress rather than perfection, you can

maintain motivation and momentum towards
your fitness aspirations.

4. Embrace Failure as a Learning Opportunity:

Failure is not a reflection of your worth or
abilities—it is simply a natural part of the
learning process. Instead of viewing failure as
a setback, reframe it as an opportunity for
growth and self-improvement. Reflect on what
went wrong, what you learned from the
experience, and how you can adjust your
approach moving forward. By embracing
failure with a growth mindset, you can turn
setbacks into stepping stones towards
success.

5. Surround Yourself with Supportive Influences:

Seek out supportive friends, family
members, or mentors who can offer
encouragement, advice, and accountability on
your fitness journey. Surrounding yourself
with positive influences can help counteract
negative self-talk and provide a sense of
belonging and validation. Additionally,
consider joining online communities or
support groups where you can connect with
like-minded individuals and share
experiences, challenges, and victories.

6. Practice Visualization and Positive Affirmations:

Visualize yourself achieving your fitness goals and imagine how it will feel to succeed. Use positive affirmations to reinforce beliefs in your abilities and reinforce a mindset of confidence and determination. Visualization and positive affirmations can help reprogram your subconscious mind and overcome limiting beliefs that may be holding you back from reaching your full potential.

In summary, overcoming mental blocks is an essential aspect of achieving success in health and fitness endeavors. By recognizing and challenging negative thoughts, cultivating self-compassion, setting realistic expectations, embracing failure as a learning opportunity, surrounding yourself with supportive influences, and practicing visualization and positive affirmations, you can break free from self-imposed limitations and unlock your true potential. With a resilient mindset and a compassionate heart, you can overcome any obstacle and achieve your health and fitness goals with confidence and determination.

Building Resilience: Cultivating a mindset of perseverance, resilience, and self-compassion on the weight loss journey.

Embarking on a weight loss journey is not just about shedding pounds—it's also about navigating the ups and downs, setbacks, and challenges that inevitably arise along the way. Building resilience— the ability to bounce back from adversity, persevere in the face of obstacles, and adapt to change—is crucial for long-term success in achieving and maintaining a healthy weight. In this chapter, we explore strategies for cultivating resilience, perseverance, and self-compassion on the weight loss journey.

1. Set Realistic Expectations:
   Unrealistic expectations can set you up for disappointment and frustration. Instead of striving for rapid weight loss or perfection, focus on setting realistic, achievable goals that are sustainable and within your control. Break larger goals into smaller, manageable steps, and celebrate each milestone along the way. By acknowledging and celebrating progress, you can maintain motivation and momentum towards your weight loss aspirations.

2. Practice Self-Compassion:

Treat yourself with kindness, understanding, and acceptance, especially during challenging times. Acknowledge that setbacks and obstacles are a natural part of the weight loss journey and respond to yourself with self-compassion rather than self-criticism. Cultivate self-care practices such as mindfulness, meditation, or spending time in nature to nurture your emotional well-being and build resilience in the face of adversity.

3. Focus on the Process, Not Just the Outcome:

While it's important to have a goal in mind, placing too much emphasis on the end result can be overwhelming and demotivating. Instead, focus on the process—the daily habits, behaviors, and choices that contribute to your overall well-being. Shift your mindset from outcome-oriented thinking to process-oriented thinking, and trust that consistent effort and dedication will lead to positive results over time.

4. Cultivate a Growth Mindset:

Embrace challenges as opportunities for growth and learning rather than viewing them as insurmountable obstacles. Adopt a growth mindset—the belief that abilities and intelligence can be developed through effort and practice—and approach setbacks with curiosity, resilience, and determination. Use failure as feedback, reflect on what you've learned, and adjust your approach accordingly.

5. Seek Support and Connection:

Surround yourself with supportive friends, family members, or mentors who can offer encouragement, advice, and accountability on your weight loss journey. Share your experiences, challenges, and victories with others who understand and empathize with your struggles. Additionally, consider joining a support group or online community where you can connect with like-minded individuals and find inspiration, motivation, and solidarity.

6. Practice Gratitude and Positive Affirmations:

Cultivate a mindset of gratitude by focusing on the positive aspects of your life and expressing appreciation for the progress you've made, no matter how small. Use positive affirmations to reinforce beliefs in your abilities and reinforce a mindset of resilience and determination. By cultivating gratitude and positivity, you can build a strong foundation for resilience and navigate the weight loss journey with grace and optimism.

In summary, building resilience is an essential aspect of achieving long-term success on the weight loss journey. By setting realistic expectations, practicing self-compassion, focusing on the process, cultivating a growth mindset, seeking support and connection, and practicing gratitude and positive affirmations, you can strengthen your ability to overcome challenges, persevere in the face of adversity, and achieve your weight loss goals with resilience and grace. With perseverance, resilience, and self-compassion as your allies, you can navigate the twists and turns of the weight loss journey with confidence and determination.

Seeking Support: Harnessing the power of community, accountability partners, and professional guidance for sustained success.

Embarking on a journey towards improved health and well-being can be both exciting and challenging. While individual motivation and determination play crucial roles, seeking support from others can significantly enhance success and sustainability. By tapping into the power of community, accountability partners, and professional guidance, individuals can gain valuable resources, encouragement, and expertise to navigate obstacles and achieve their goals. In this chapter, we explore the importance of seeking support and strategies for harnessing its transformative potential.

1. Community Connection:

Joining a community of like-minded individuals who share similar health and wellness goals can provide invaluable support, motivation, and camaraderie. Whether through local fitness groups, online forums, social media communities, or support groups, connecting with others who understand and empathize with your journey can foster a sense of belonging and solidarity. Sharing experiences, challenges, and successes with a supportive community can inspire and motivate you to stay committed to your health goals.

2. Accountability Partners:

Accountability partners serve as trusted allies who provide encouragement, accountability, and mutual support on the journey towards improved health and well-being. Whether it's a friend, family member, or coworker, having someone to share your goals with and hold you accountable can significantly increase your likelihood of success. Schedule regular check-ins, set shared goals, and celebrate each other's progress to maintain motivation and momentum.

3. Professional Guidance:

Seeking guidance from qualified professionals, such as registered dietitians, personal trainers, health coaches, or therapists, can provide personalized support and expertise tailored to your specific needs and goals. Professional guidance can help you develop a customized nutrition plan, create an effective workout routine, overcome mental and emotional barriers, and navigate complex health issues. Working with a professional can offer clarity, direction, and accountability on your journey towards improved health and well-being.

4. Group Programs and Workshops:

Participating in group programs, workshops, or classes led by experienced professionals can offer structured guidance, support, and accountability in a supportive group setting. Whether it's a weight loss program, fitness challenge, cooking class, or mindfulness workshop, group settings provide opportunities for learning, growth, and connection with others who share similar goals and aspirations. Group programs can offer a sense of camaraderie, accountability, and shared progress that fuels motivation and fosters success.

5. Online Resources and Tools:

In today's digital age, a wealth of online resources and tools are available to support individuals on their health and wellness journey. From educational articles and videos to meal planning apps, workout trackers, and virtual coaching platforms, online resources offer convenient and accessible support tailored to individual preferences and needs. Take advantage of online communities, webinars, and digital platforms to access information, inspiration, and guidance from experts and peers alike.

6. Cultivate a Supportive Environment:

Surround yourself with individuals, environments, and resources that support your health and wellness goals. Communicate your intentions and boundaries with friends, family members, and coworkers, and enlist their support in creating a supportive environment that nurtures your well-being. Surround yourself with positive influences, set boundaries around negative influences, and

prioritize self-care activities that replenish
your energy and resilience.

In summary, seeking support from
community, accountability partners, and
professional guidance can amplify your efforts
towards improved health and well-being. By
tapping into the collective wisdom,
encouragement, and resources available
through supportive networks and expert
guidance, you can overcome obstacles, stay
motivated, and achieve lasting success on
your journey towards a healthier, happier life.
With the power of support and collaboration,
your health goals become not just aspirations,
but achievable realities.

Chapter 5: Sleep, Stress, and Self-Care

Prioritizing Sleep: Exploring the link between quality sleep, metabolism, and weight management.

In our quest for improved health and well-being, we often focus on nutrition and exercise while overlooking the critical role of sleep. However, quality sleep is essential for overall health, and its impact on metabolism and weight management cannot be overstated. In this chapter, we delve into the intricate relationship between sleep, metabolism, and weight management, and explore strategies for prioritizing sleep to support optimal health outcomes.

1. The Sleep-Metabolism Connection:
Sleep plays a fundamental role in regulating various physiological processes, including metabolism, appetite regulation, and energy balance. Research has shown that inadequate or poor-quality sleep can disrupt hormonal balance, leading to alterations in appetite-regulating hormones such as leptin and

ghrelin. These hormonal imbalances can increase hunger and cravings for high-calorie, carbohydrate-rich foods, leading to overeating and weight gain over time.

2. Impact on Metabolic Health:

Quality sleep is crucial for maintaining metabolic health and insulin sensitivity—the body's ability to regulate blood sugar levels. Chronic sleep deprivation or sleep disturbances have been associated with insulin resistance, impaired glucose tolerance, and an increased risk of type 2 diabetes. Additionally, inadequate sleep can disrupt circadian rhythms, which play a role in regulating metabolism, energy expenditure, and nutrient partitioning.

3. Influence on Weight Management:

The relationship between sleep and weight management is bidirectional, with sleep quality and duration influencing weight status, and vice versa. Studies have shown that individuals who consistently get inadequate sleep are more likely to be overweight or obese compared to those who get sufficient sleep. Poor sleep quality can also compromise efforts towards weight loss by affecting appetite regulation, food choices, and energy expenditure.

4. Strategies for Prioritizing Sleep:

Recognizing the importance of sleep for overall health and weight management, it's essential to prioritize sleep as part of a comprehensive wellness strategy. Here are some strategies for improving sleep quality and duration:

- *Establish a Consistent Sleep Schedule*: Go to bed and wake up at the same time every day, even on weekends, to regulate your body's internal clock.

- *Create a Relaxing Bedtime Routine*: Develop a relaxing pre-sleep routine to signal to your body that it's time to wind down. This may include activities such as reading, gentle stretching, meditation, or taking a warm bath.

- *Create a Sleep-Conducive Environment*: Make your bedroom a comfortable, quiet, and dark environment conducive to sleep. Invest in a comfortable mattress and pillows, and consider using blackout curtains or white noise machines to block out distractions.

- *Limit Stimulants and Electronics Before Bed*: Avoid stimulants such as caffeine and nicotine in the hours leading up to bedtime, and minimize exposure to electronic devices such as smartphones, tablets, and computers, which emit blue light that can interfere with sleep.

- Practice Stress Reduction Techniques: Manage stress and anxiety through relaxation techniques such as deep breathing, progressive muscle relaxation, or mindfulness meditation to promote relaxation and improve sleep quality.

By prioritizing sleep and adopting healthy sleep habits, you can support metabolic health, regulate appetite and weight, and optimize overall well-being. Incorporating quality sleep as a cornerstone of your health routine can yield profound benefits for both body and mind, enhancing your resilience, vitality, and quality of life.

Stress Management Strategies: Techniques for reducing stress levels, managing cortisol, and preventing emotional eating.

In today's fast-paced world, stress has become a common part of everyday life, often taking a toll on both our physical and mental well-being. Chronic stress can lead to elevated levels of cortisol, the body's primary stress hormone, which has been linked to a variety of health issues, including weight gain and emotional eating. In this chapter, we explore effective stress management strategies to reduce stress levels, regulate cortisol production, and prevent emotional eating.

1. Mindfulness Meditation:

Mindfulness meditation is a powerful practice for reducing stress and promoting emotional well-being. By focusing attention on the present moment without judgment, mindfulness meditation can help cultivate a sense of calm, clarity, and inner peace. Regular practice of mindfulness meditation has been shown to reduce cortisol levels, lower blood pressure, and improve mood and resilience in the face of stress.

2. Deep Breathing Exercises:

Deep breathing exercises, such as diaphragmatic breathing or belly breathing, can activate the body's relaxation response and help reduce stress levels. By slowing down the breath and engaging the diaphragm, deep breathing promotes relaxation, lowers heart rate, and decreases cortisol production. Practice deep breathing exercises regularly, especially during times of heightened stress or anxiety, to induce a state of calm and balance.

3. Regular Physical Activity:

Engaging in regular physical activity is an effective way to combat stress and promote overall well-being. Exercise has been shown to stimulate the release of endorphins, the body's natural mood-enhancing chemicals, while also reducing cortisol levels. Whether it's a brisk walk, a yoga class, or a high-intensity workout, find physical activities that you enjoy and incorporate them into your daily routine to help manage stress and improve resilience.

4. Prioritize Sleep:

Quality sleep is essential for stress management and overall health. Chronic sleep deprivation can disrupt cortisol regulation, leading to elevated stress levels and impaired cognitive function. Aim for 7-9 hours of quality sleep per night and establish a relaxing bedtime routine to promote restful sleep. Create a comfortable sleep environment, limit exposure to screens before bed, and practice relaxation techniques to wind down and prepare for sleep.

5. Healthy Nutrition:

Nutrition plays a key role in stress management, as certain foods and nutrients can influence cortisol levels and mood. Focus on eating a balanced diet rich in whole, nutrient-dense foods such as fruits,

vegetables, lean proteins, and healthy fats.
Avoid excessive caffeine and sugar, which can
contribute to cortisol spikes and exacerbate
stress levels. Stay hydrated and prioritize
regular meals and snacks to maintain stable
blood sugar levels and support optimal energy
levels throughout the day.

6. Cultivate Supportive Relationships:

Strong social connections and support
networks are essential for coping with stress
and building resilience. Reach out to friends,
family members, or support groups for
emotional support and encouragement during
times of stress. Share your feelings and
experiences with trusted individuals who can
offer empathy, perspective, and practical
advice. Cultivate meaningful relationships
that provide a sense of belonging, connection,
and validation.

By incorporating these stress management
strategies into your daily routine, you can
reduce stress levels, regulate cortisol
production, and prevent emotional eating.
Prioritize self-care, relaxation, and healthy
coping mechanisms to build resilience and
foster a sense of calm, balance, and well-being
in your life. Remember that managing stress
is a lifelong journey, and it's okay to seek

professional support if you need additional help or guidance along the way.

Self-Care Rituals: Nurturing the body and mind through relaxation, mindfulness, and holistic wellness practices.

In our fast-paced and often hectic lives, it's essential to prioritize self-care as a means of maintaining balance, reducing stress, and promoting overall well-being. Self-care rituals are intentional practices that nourish the body, mind, and spirit, fostering a sense of peace, rejuvenation, and inner harmony. In this chapter, we explore various self-care rituals that promote relaxation, mindfulness, and holistic wellness.

1. Mindful Movement:
   Engaging in mindful movement practices such as yoga, tai chi, or qigong can help cultivate a deeper connection between the body and mind. These gentle, flowing movements promote flexibility, strength, and balance while also encouraging mindfulness and presence in the moment. Incorporate mindful movement into your daily routine to

release tension, reduce stress, and enhance overall well-being.

2. Relaxation Techniques:

Relaxation techniques such as deep breathing, progressive muscle relaxation, or guided imagery can help induce a state of relaxation and calm the nervous system. Take time each day to practice relaxation techniques, either through structured exercises or simply by finding moments of stillness and quietude. Cultivate an environment conducive to relaxation, whether it's a cozy corner of your home, a peaceful nature setting, or a soothing bath with essential oils and candles.

3. Mindfulness Meditation:

Mindfulness meditation is a powerful practice for cultivating present-moment awareness and fostering a sense of inner peace and tranquility. Set aside time each day for mindfulness meditation, even if it's just a few minutes of focused attention on the breath or body sensations. Incorporate mindfulness into everyday activities such as eating, walking, or washing dishes, bringing awareness and intention to each moment with curiosity and non-judgment.

4. Holistic Wellness Practices:

Holistic wellness practices encompass a wide range of modalities that address the interconnectedness of the body, mind, and spirit. Explore holistic wellness practices such as aromatherapy, massage therapy, acupuncture, or energy healing to promote balance and harmony within the body. Experiment with different modalities to discover what resonates with you and incorporate them into your self-care routine as needed.

5. Nourishing Nutrition:

Nourishing your body with wholesome, nutrient-dense foods is an essential aspect of self-care. Prioritize a balanced diet rich in fruits, vegetables, whole grains, lean proteins, and healthy fats to support optimal health and well-being. Pay attention to how different foods make you feel and cultivate mindful eating habits that honor your body's nutritional needs and preferences.

6. Creative Expression:

Engaging in creative expression is a powerful form of self-care that allows you to tap into your inner creativity and self-expression. Whether it's painting, writing, music, dance, or crafting, find ways to express yourself creatively and nurture your artistic side. Creativity can be a source of joy, inspiration, and self-discovery, providing an outlet for emotions and a means of connecting with your innermost desires and passions.

7. Connection with Nature:

Spending time in nature is a potent form of self-care that nourishes the body, mind, and spirit. Take time to immerse yourself in the natural world, whether it's going for a hike, gardening, or simply sitting outside and soaking up the sights, sounds, and smells of the outdoors. Nature has a calming and grounding effect that can help reduce stress, boost mood, and promote a sense of interconnectedness with the world around you.

Incorporating self-care rituals into your daily routine is a powerful way to prioritize your health, happiness, and well-being. Experiment with different practices and find what resonates with you, creating a personalized self-care routine that nourishes your body, mind, and spirit. Remember that self-care is not selfish—it's an essential aspect of maintaining balance and vitality in all areas of your life.

Chapter 6: Embracing Change for Long-Term Success

Sustainable Habits: Building lasting habits that support a healthy lifestyle, rather than quick-fix solutions.

In the quest for improved health and well-being, it's essential to prioritize sustainable habits—lifestyle practices that can be maintained over the long term and contribute to lasting health outcomes. While quick-fix solutions may offer temporary results, sustainable habits provide a solid foundation for ongoing health and vitality. In this chapter, we explore the importance of sustainable habits and strategies for building practices that support a healthy lifestyle.

1. Focus on Consistency Over Perfection: Sustainable habits are built through consistent, incremental progress rather than dramatic, short-term changes. Instead of striving for perfection or instant results, focus on making small, manageable changes to your

daily routine that you can maintain over time. Celebrate each small victory and view setbacks as opportunities for growth and learning rather than reasons to give up.

2. Set Realistic and Achievable Goals:

When establishing new habits, set realistic and achievable goals that align with your values, priorities, and lifestyle. Break larger goals into smaller, actionable steps, and focus on making gradual progress towards your objectives. By setting attainable goals, you'll build confidence, momentum, and motivation to sustain your efforts over the long term.

3. Find Enjoyable Activities:

Sustainable habits are more likely to stick when they're enjoyable and align with your interests and preferences. Experiment with different forms of exercise, nutritious foods, and self-care practices to discover what resonates with you. Choose activities that bring you joy, satisfaction, and fulfillment, making it easier to incorporate them into your daily routine and maintain them over time.

4. Prioritize Balance and Flexibility:

Sustainable habits prioritize balance and flexibility, allowing for occasional indulgences and deviations from the routine without derailing progress. Avoid rigid rules or restrictive diets that can lead to feelings of deprivation and burnout. Instead, practice moderation, portion control, and mindful eating, allowing yourself to enjoy your favorite foods in moderation while also nourishing your body with nutritious choices.

5. Cultivate Self-Compassion:

Building sustainable habits requires patience, resilience, and self-compassion. Be kind to yourself and acknowledge that change takes time and effort. Embrace the process of self-improvement with curiosity, openness, and a willingness to learn from both successes and setbacks. Treat yourself with the same kindness and understanding that you would offer to a friend facing similar challenges.

6. Create Supportive Environments:

Surround yourself with environments, influences, and relationships that support your efforts towards building sustainable habits. Seek out social support, accountability partners, and positive role models who can offer encouragement, guidance, and motivation along the way. Create environments that make healthy choices the default option, whether it's stocking your kitchen with nutritious foods, scheduling

regular exercise sessions, or setting
boundaries around screen time and sleep.

7. Practice Mindfulness and Reflection:

Cultivate mindfulness and self-awareness by
regularly reflecting on your habits, behaviors,
and choices. Notice how different activities
make you feel physically, mentally, and
emotionally, and adjust your habits
accordingly. Pay attention to triggers,
patterns, and obstacles that may hinder
progress, and brainstorm alternative
strategies for overcoming challenges and
staying on track.

In summary, building sustainable habits is a
gradual, iterative process that requires
patience, perseverance, and self-compassion.
By focusing on consistency over perfection,
setting realistic goals, finding enjoyable
activities, prioritizing balance and flexibility,
cultivating self-compassion, creating
supportive environments, and practicing
mindfulness and reflection, you can build
lasting practices that support a healthy,
fulfilling lifestyle. Remember that sustainable
habits are not a destination but a journey—a
journey towards greater health, happiness,
and well-being that unfolds one step at a time.

Celebrating Progress: Recognizing milestones, victories, and non-scale achievements along the way.

Embarking on a journey towards weight loss is akin to embarking on an odyssey—a quest filled with challenges, triumphs, and transformative moments. Amidst the ups and downs of this journey, it's crucial to take pause and celebrate the progress you've made, regardless of the number on the scale. Here, we delve into the significance of recognizing milestones, victories, and non-scale achievements along the way.

1. Embracing Non-Scale Victories
Weight loss is not solely about the digits on the scale; it encompasses a myriad of non-scale victories that signify profound changes in your health and well-being. These victories might manifest as increased energy levels, improved mood, enhanced sleep quality, or heightened self-confidence. Embrace and celebrate these non-scale victories as tangible evidence of your progress and resilience.

2. Milestones Worth Celebrating
Setting and celebrating milestones along your journey provides direction and motivation, guiding you towards your ultimate goals.

Whether it's reaching a specific weight loss target, fitting into a smaller clothing size, or mastering a new fitness challenge, each milestone represents a significant step forward. Take time to acknowledge and celebrate these milestones as markers of your dedication and perseverance.

3. Victories Beyond the Scale

Beyond the realm of weight loss, victories abound in various facets of your life. Improved fitness levels, healthier eating habits, increased flexibility, or enhanced mental clarity are victories worthy of celebration. Recognize the holistic benefits of your efforts and celebrate the positive changes that extend beyond mere numbers on the scale. These victories reflect your commitment to overall well-being and self-improvement.

4. Cultivating a Culture of Celebration

Foster an environment that celebrates progress and success, both individually and collectively. Surround yourself with supportive friends, family members, or accountability partners who cheer you on and celebrate your victories with you. Share your milestones and achievements with your community, whether it's through social media, support groups, or wellness forums. Cultivate a culture of

celebration that uplifts and inspires you on
your journey.

5. The Power of Reflection and Gratitude
Reflection and gratitude are potent tools for
recognizing and celebrating progress. Take
time to reflect on how far you've come, the
obstacles you've overcome, and the lessons
you've learned along the way. Express
gratitude for the resilience, determination, and
support that have fueled your journey.
Celebrate the growth, both personal and
physical, that you've experienced, and honor
the transformative power of your efforts.

In conclusion, celebrating progress is not just
about acknowledging achievements—it's about
honoring the journey, embracing the process,
and cultivating a mindset of gratitude and
resilience. So, as you navigate your weight
loss journey, remember to celebrate every
milestone, victory, and non-scale achievement
along the way. Each step forward is a triumph
worth celebrating, bringing you closer to a
healthier, happier, and more fulfilled version
of yourself.

Staying Motivated: Renewing commitment, adjusting strategies, and staying resilient in the face of setbacks.

Maintaining motivation throughout your weight loss journey is often likened to a marathon rather than a sprint—it requires perseverance, adaptability, and a steadfast commitment to your goals. In this section, we delve into the strategies for staying motivated, renewing your commitment, adjusting your approach, and cultivating resilience in the face of setbacks.

1. Renewing Commitment to Your Goals
Periodically reassessing and reaffirming your commitment to your weight loss goals is essential for staying motivated and focused. Take time to revisit your reasons for embarking on this journey, whether it's to improve your health, boost your confidence, or enhance your quality of life. Visualize the outcomes you aspire to achieve and reaffirm your dedication to making them a reality. Remember that your goals are worth pursuing, and your commitment is the driving force behind your success.

2. Adjusting Strategies for Success

Flexibility and adaptability are key attributes of successful weight loss journeys. If you encounter obstacles or plateaus along the way, it may be necessary to adjust your strategies and tactics accordingly. Reflect on what's working well and what could be improved, and be open to experimenting with new approaches. Whether it's modifying your exercise routine, fine-tuning your nutrition plan, or seeking support from a health professional, be proactive in adapting your strategies to align with your evolving needs and circumstances.

3. Cultivating Resilience in the Face of Setbacks

Setbacks and challenges are inevitable on any journey towards personal growth and transformation. When faced with setbacks, it's crucial to cultivate resilience—the ability to bounce back, learn from setbacks, and continue moving forward despite adversity. Instead of viewing setbacks as failures, reframe them as opportunities for growth and learning. Reflect on the lessons you've gleaned from setbacks, and draw upon your inner strength and determination to overcome obstacles and persevere towards your goals.

4. Finding Inspiration and Support

Surrounding yourself with sources of inspiration and support can bolster your motivation and resilience on your weight loss journey. Seek out role models, success stories, or motivational quotes that resonate with you and remind you of the possibilities that lie ahead. Engage with supportive communities, whether it's through online forums, support groups, or wellness programs, where you can connect with like-minded individuals who understand and encourage your journey. Remember that you're not alone on this path, and drawing upon the strength and support of others can help fuel your motivation and resilience.

5. Celebrating Progress Along the Way

Finally, don't forget to celebrate your progress and achievements along the way. Acknowledge and celebrate every milestone, victory, and non-scale achievement, no matter how small. Celebrating progress reinforces your sense of accomplishment, boosts your morale, and fuels your motivation to continue pushing forward. Take time to reflect on how far you've come, and let each success serve as a reminder of your strength, determination, and unwavering commitment to your goals.

In conclusion, staying motivated on your weight loss journey requires dedication, adaptability, and resilience. By renewing your commitment to your goals, adjusting your strategies as needed, cultivating resilience in the face of setbacks, seeking inspiration and support, and celebrating progress along the way, you can stay motivated and focused on your path towards health, happiness, and well-being. Remember that every step forward, no matter how small, brings you closer to achieving your goals and living the vibrant, fulfilling life you deserve.

Chapter 7: Beyond Weight Loss: Thriving in a Healthier Body and Mind

Holistic Wellness: Integrating physical, mental, and emotional well-being into everyday life.

Achieving optimal health and well-being goes beyond the physical realm—it encompasses the integration of physical, mental, and emotional wellness into every aspect of your life. In this section, we explore the principles of holistic wellness and provide practical strategies for nurturing your overall well-being.

1. Understanding Holistic Wellness
Holistic wellness is a comprehensive approach to health that acknowledges the interconnectedness of the body, mind, and spirit. It recognizes that physical health, mental clarity, emotional resilience, and spiritual fulfillment are all intertwined and influence one another. Rather than treating symptoms in isolation, holistic wellness addresses the root causes of imbalances and

seeks to restore harmony and vitality on all levels.

2. Nurturing Physical Well-being

Physical well-being encompasses more than just diet and exercise—it encompasses all aspects of physical health, including nutrition, movement, sleep, and self-care. Prioritize nourishing your body with wholesome, nutrient-dense foods, staying active through regular exercise and movement, prioritizing quality sleep, and practicing self-care activities that promote relaxation and rejuvenation. Listen to your body's cues and honor its needs with compassion and care.

3. Cultivating Mental Clarity and Focus

Mental well-being involves cultivating clarity, focus, and resilience in the face of life's challenges. Practice mindfulness and meditation to quiet the mind and cultivate present-moment awareness. Engage in activities that stimulate your intellect and creativity, such as reading, learning new skills, or engaging in hobbies. Set boundaries around technology and media consumption to protect your mental space and promote mental clarity.

4. Honoring Emotional Resilience and
   Self-Compassion

Emotional well-being entails acknowledging and processing your emotions in healthy ways, fostering resilience, and cultivating self-compassion. Practice emotional self-awareness by tuning into your feelings and acknowledging them without judgment. Develop healthy coping strategies for managing stress, such as deep breathing, journaling, or talking to a trusted friend or therapist. Cultivate self-compassion by treating yourself with kindness and understanding, especially during challenging times.

5. Fostering Spiritual Fulfillment and
   Connection

Spiritual well-being involves finding meaning, purpose, and connection in life, whether through religion, nature, relationships, or personal values. Nurture your spiritual health by engaging in practices that align with your beliefs and values, such as prayer, meditation, or spending time in nature. Cultivate gratitude and appreciation for the beauty and wonder of life, and seek out opportunities for connection and community with others who share your spiritual beliefs.

6. Integrating Holistic Wellness into
    Everyday Life

Integrating holistic wellness into your everyday life involves making conscious choices that support your overall well-being in every aspect of your daily routine. Set aside time each day for self-care activities, such as exercise, meditation, or creative expression. Prioritize nourishing your body with healthy foods, staying hydrated, and getting enough sleep. Seek out activities and experiences that bring you joy, fulfillment, and a sense of connection with yourself and others.

In conclusion, holistic wellness is about nurturing your body, mind, and spirit in harmony to achieve optimal health and well-being. By integrating physical, mental, and emotional wellness into your everyday life and making conscious choices that support your overall well-being, you can cultivate a vibrant, fulfilling life that honors your holistic health and vitality. Remember that wellness is a journey, not a destination, and each step you take towards nurturing your holistic well-being brings you closer to living your best life.

Body Positivity and Self-Love: Fostering acceptance, gratitude, and appreciation for the body's journey and capabilities.

Embracing body positivity and cultivating self-love are integral aspects of holistic well-being, essential for nurturing a healthy relationship with your body and fostering a sense of acceptance, gratitude, and appreciation for its journey and capabilities. In this section, we delve into the principles of body positivity and self-love and provide practical strategies for integrating them into your daily life.

1. Embracing Body Positivity
Body positivity is a movement that celebrates diversity, challenges societal beauty standards, and promotes acceptance and respect for all bodies, regardless of shape, size, or appearance. Embracing body positivity involves shifting your focus from unrealistic ideals to appreciating the uniqueness and beauty of your own body. Practice self-compassion and kindness towards yourself, and cultivate a mindset of acceptance and gratitude for your body's inherent worth and resilience.

2. Cultivating Self-Love
Self-love is the foundation of a healthy
relationship with your body and encompasses
nurturing compassion, acceptance, and
appreciation for yourself as a whole.
Cultivating self-love involves recognizing and
challenging negative self-talk and limiting
beliefs about your body, replacing them with
affirming and empowering thoughts. Practice
acts of self-care and self-kindness, such as
speaking to yourself with kindness, engaging
in activities that bring you joy and fulfillment,
and prioritizing your well-being in all aspects
of your life.

3. Practicing Gratitude for Your Body
Gratitude is a powerful practice that fosters
appreciation for the body's journey and
capabilities. Take time each day to express
gratitude for your body and all that it allows
you to do, whether it's moving, breathing,
sensing, or experiencing life's joys. Focus on
the functionality and resilience of your body
rather than its appearance, and acknowledge
the incredible feats it performs each day to
support you in living a full and vibrant life.

4. Honoring Your Body's Journey
Your body is a testament to the journey you've
traveled—a journey marked by growth,
resilience, and transformation. Honor and

celebrate your body's journey, recognizing the strength, wisdom, and beauty it has gained along the way. Embrace the changes and fluctuations that naturally occur as a part of life's ebbs and flows, and view them as symbols of your body's adaptability and resilience in navigating life's challenges and triumphs.

5. Engaging in Body-Positive Practices

Engage in practices and activities that promote body positivity and self-love, such as surrounding yourself with positive influences, consuming media that celebrates diverse bodies, and participating in body-positive communities and events. Challenge societal norms and messages that perpetuate unrealistic beauty standards, and advocate for inclusivity, diversity, and acceptance in all areas of life. Remember that every act of self-love and body positivity contributes to a culture of acceptance and empowerment for yourself and others.

6. Affirming Your Worth and Value

Above all, affirm your worth and value as a unique and valuable individual, regardless of your body's appearance or perceived flaws. Recognize that your worth is not determined by external factors, but by your inherent dignity, humanity, and capacity for love and connection. Treat yourself with the same kindness, compassion, and respect that you would offer to a cherished friend or loved one, and affirm your worthiness of love, acceptance, and happiness exactly as you are.

In conclusion, embracing body positivity and cultivating self-love are essential components of holistic well-being, vital for nurturing a healthy relationship with your body and fostering acceptance, gratitude, and appreciation for its journey and capabilities. By embracing body positivity, practicing self-love, cultivating gratitude for your body, honoring its journey, engaging in body-positive practices, and affirming your worth and value, you can cultivate a deep sense of acceptance, empowerment, and joy in your relationship with your body and yourself.

Inspiring Others: Paying it forward by sharing knowledge, supporting others, and contributing to a culture of health and empowerment.

Inspiring others is a powerful way to give back and contribute to a culture of health, wellness, and empowerment. By sharing your knowledge, supporting others on their journeys, and fostering a community of encouragement and positivity, you can create a ripple effect that uplifts and empowers those around you. In this section, we explore the importance of inspiring others and provide practical strategies for paying it forward.

1. Sharing Knowledge and Expertise
One of the most impactful ways to inspire others is by sharing your knowledge and expertise. Whether you've achieved success in your own weight loss journey, mastered healthy habits, or gained insights into nutrition and fitness, your experience can be invaluable to others who are on a similar path. Share your journey, tips, and strategies through blogs, social media, workshops, or community events, and empower others with the knowledge and tools they need to succeed.

2. Supporting Others on Their Journeys
Support is a cornerstone of success on the weight loss journey, and offering encouragement, guidance, and empathy to others can make a world of difference. Be a supportive presence for friends, family members, or community members who are navigating their own health and wellness journeys. Listen with empathy, offer words of encouragement, and provide practical support, such as accountability check-ins, workout buddies, or meal prep assistance.

Your support can be a lifeline for others as they navigate the ups and downs of their journey.

3. Leading by Example

Leading by example is a powerful way to inspire others to prioritize their health and well-being. Model healthy behaviors, such as nutritious eating, regular exercise, stress management, and self-care practices, in your own life, and let your actions speak louder than words. Show others that prioritizing health and wellness is achievable, enjoyable, and rewarding, and inspire them to follow suit by witnessing the positive impact it has on your life.

4. Fostering a Culture of Health and Empowerment

Contribute to a culture of health and empowerment within your community by fostering an environment that values and supports well-being. Advocate for policies and initiatives that promote access to healthy food, safe spaces for physical activity, and resources for mental health and wellness. Create or participate in community events, support groups, or wellness programs that provide opportunities for education, connection, and empowerment. By working together to create a culture of health, you can inspire and empower others to prioritize their well-being and thrive.

5. Celebrating Successes and Milestones
Celebrate the successes and milestones of others with genuine enthusiasm and joy. Whether it's a friend reaching a weight loss goal, mastering a new fitness challenge, or adopting healthier habits, take time to acknowledge and celebrate their achievements. Your support and encouragement can bolster their confidence, motivation, and sense of accomplishment, reinforcing their commitment to their health and well-being.

6. Paying It Forward with Gratitude
Finally, pay it forward with gratitude by expressing appreciation for those who have inspired and supported you on your own journey. Take time to thank mentors, role models, friends, or loved ones who have encouraged and empowered you along the way. By acknowledging the impact they've had on your life, you not only honor their contributions but also perpetuate a cycle of gratitude, kindness, and inspiration that uplifts and enriches the lives of others.

In conclusion, inspiring others is a meaningful way to contribute to a culture of health, wellness, and empowerment. By sharing your knowledge, supporting others on their journeys, leading by example, fostering a culture of health and empowerment, celebrating successes, and paying it forward with gratitude, you can create a ripple effect of positivity and inspiration that transforms lives and communities. Remember that every act of kindness, encouragement, and support has the power to make a difference in the lives of others, and by inspiring others, you can be a catalyst for positive change in the world.

Reflecting on personal growth, resilience, and achievements on the weight loss journey.

Embarking on a weight loss journey is not just about shedding pounds—it's also a profound journey of personal growth, resilience, and self-discovery. Along the way, individuals encounter challenges, setbacks, and victories that shape their understanding of themselves and their capacity for change. In this chapter, we explore the importance of reflecting on personal growth, resilience, and achievements on the weight loss journey, and how these insights can empower individuals to continue progressing towards their goals.

1. Celebrating Progress:

Reflecting on personal growth and achievements involves acknowledging and celebrating progress, no matter how small. Take time to recognize the positive changes you've made—whether it's adopting healthier eating habits, increasing physical activity, or overcoming mental barriers. Celebrate milestones, such as reaching a certain weight loss goal, fitting into a smaller clothing size, or completing a challenging workout, as markers of your progress and perseverance.

2. Cultivating Resilience:

The weight loss journey is often accompanied by setbacks, obstacles, and moments of doubt. Reflecting on personal resilience involves recognizing your ability to bounce back from challenges, learn from setbacks, and keep moving forward. Identify times when you've faced adversity and overcome it with determination, perseverance, and resilience. These experiences build inner strength and confidence that can sustain you through future challenges on your journey.

3. Recognizing Non-Scale Victories:

While weight loss is a common measure of success on the weight loss journey, it's essential to recognize and celebrate non-scale victories as well. Reflect on the positive changes beyond the number on the scale—such as increased energy levels, improved mood, better sleep quality, and enhanced self-confidence. These non-scale victories are often more meaningful indicators of overall health and well-being than weight alone.

4. Acknowledging Inner Growth:

Reflecting on personal growth involves acknowledging the internal transformations that occur on the weight loss journey. Consider how your mindset, attitudes, and beliefs about yourself and your body have evolved throughout the process. Have you developed greater self-awareness, self-compassion, or self-confidence? Have you challenged limiting beliefs or negative self-talk? Recognize the inner growth that accompanies physical transformation and celebrate the person you are becoming.

5. Learning from Setbacks:

Setbacks and challenges are inevitable on any journey towards personal growth and self-improvement. Reflect on times when you've faced obstacles or setbacks on your weight loss journey and consider what lessons you've learned from these experiences. What strategies helped you overcome obstacles?

What insights have you gained about your strengths, weaknesses, and areas for growth? Use setbacks as opportunities for learning, growth, and refinement of your approach.

6. Practicing Gratitude:

Reflecting on personal growth, resilience, and achievements involves cultivating an attitude of gratitude for the progress you've made and the support you've received along the way. Take time to express gratitude for your body's resilience, your ability to overcome challenges, and the support of friends, family, or professionals who have helped you on your journey. Gratitude cultivates a positive mindset and fosters resilience in the face of adversity.

In summary, reflecting on personal growth, resilience, and achievements on the weight loss journey is a powerful practice that fosters self-awareness, gratitude, and empowerment. By celebrating progress, cultivating resilience, recognizing non-scale victories, acknowledging inner growth, learning from setbacks, and practicing gratitude, individuals can gain valuable insights and motivation to continue moving forward towards their health and wellness goals. Reflecting on the journey not only honors how far you've come but also

provides clarity and inspiration for the road
ahead.

Conclusion: Looking ahead and embracing a future of vitality, balance, and fulfillment

As we reflect on our health and wellness journey thus far, we are filled with gratitude for the progress we've made, the lessons we've learned, and the growth we've experienced. Looking ahead to the future, we are filled with excitement and anticipation for what lies ahead—a future filled with vitality, balance, and fulfillment.

1. Embracing Vitality:

Looking ahead, we envision a future filled with vitality—a state of vibrant health, energy, and vitality that allows us to fully engage in life's adventures and pursuits. We commit to nourishing our bodies with wholesome foods, staying active, and prioritizing self-care practices that promote physical, mental, and emotional well-being. We embrace the joy of movement, the beauty of nature, and the gift of vitality that allows us to live life to the fullest.

2. Cultivating Balance:

In the future, we strive to cultivate balance in all aspects of our lives—balancing work and play, rest and activity, and commitments and leisure time. We recognize the importance of setting boundaries, prioritizing self-care, and creating space for relaxation and rejuvenation. We seek harmony in our relationships, our schedules, and our environments, fostering a sense of equilibrium that nourishes our souls and fuels our passions.

3. Pursuing Fulfillment:

Looking ahead, we aspire to pursue fulfillment—a sense of purpose, meaning, and satisfaction that enriches our lives and brings us joy. We commit to following our passions, pursuing our dreams, and living authentically in alignment with our values and beliefs. We embrace opportunities for growth, learning, and self-discovery, knowing that true fulfillment comes from within and is cultivated through intentional living and mindful choices.

4. Embracing Change and Adaptation:

As we look to the future, we recognize that change is inevitable and that adaptation is key to navigating life's twists and turns. We embrace change as an opportunity for growth, resilience, and transformation, knowing that each new challenge presents an opportunity for learning and evolution. We approach the future with optimism, curiosity, and a willingness to embrace the unknown, confident in our ability to navigate whatever lies ahead with grace and resilience.

5. Fostering Connection and Community:

In the future, we cherish the importance of fostering connection and community—building meaningful relationships, supporting one another, and contributing to the well-being of those around us. We value the power of human connection to uplift, inspire, and unite us in our shared journey towards health, happiness, and fulfillment. We commit to nurturing our relationships, both online and offline, and to fostering a sense of belonging and solidarity within our communities.

6. Living with Gratitude and Presence:

Looking ahead, we commit to living with gratitude and presence—cultivating an attitude of appreciation for the abundance and beauty that surrounds us, and savoring each moment with mindfulness and awareness. We recognize that life is a precious gift, and we vow to live each day with intention, purpose, and gratitude, knowing that each moment is an opportunity to create a life of meaning, joy, and fulfillment.

As we embrace a future of vitality, balance, and fulfillment, we are filled with hope, optimism, and excitement for the journey ahead. We commit to nurturing our health and well-being, fostering connection and community, and living with gratitude, presence, and intention each step of the way. Together, we embark on this journey with open hearts and minds, ready to embrace whatever the future may hold with courage, resilience, and a sense of wonder.

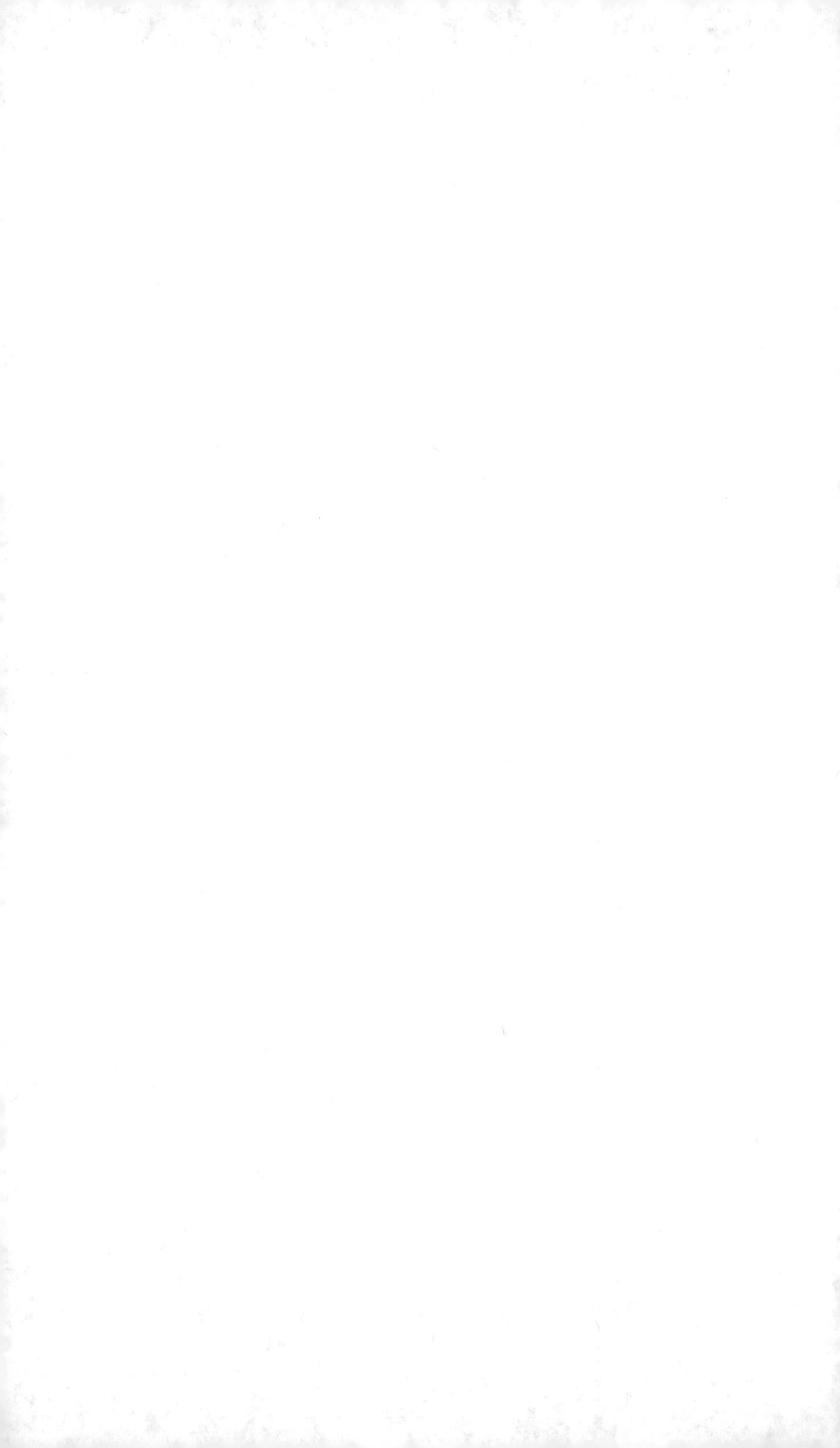